JANE ELLIOTT

Play Therapy for Autism

First edition

This book was professionally typeset on Reedsy.
Find out more at reedsy.com

Contents

1

Understanding Autism

Autism Spectrum Disorder (ASD) is a condition that impacts communication, social interaction, and behavior, and arises from atypical neurodevelopment. It is a spectrum disorder, meaning that the severity of symptoms can vary widely from person to person.

Symptoms of ASD typically appear in early childhood, and some of the most common signs include delayed speech and language development, difficulty with social interaction, and repetitive behaviors or restricted interests.

The prevalence of ASD has increased in recent years, with the Centers for Disease Control and Prevention (CDC) estimating that approximately 1 in 54 children in the United States have ASD.

Although the precise reasons behind ASD are not yet completely comprehended, investigations propose that a blend of hereditary and environmental elements could play a role in the onset of the condition.

Currently, there is no cure for ASD, but early diagnosis and intervention can help children with ASD develop the skills they need to communicate, socialize, and function more effectively. Treatment for ASD may involve a variety of therapies, including behavioral therapy, speech therapy, and occupational therapy.

In recent years, the use of play therapy techniques in the treatment of ASD has gained increasing attention. Play therapy involves using toys, games, and other play-based activities to help children develop social, emotional, and cognitive skills.

Research has shown that play therapy can be an effective treatment for children with ASD, helping to improve communication, socialization, and behavior. In the following chapters, we will explore the use of play therapy techniques in the treatment of ASD, including specific techniques and strategies for incorporating play into ASD therapy sessions.

We will also discuss the benefits of parental involvement in play therapy, the role of creative arts therapy in ASD treatment, and the future of play therapy for autism.

It is important to note that while play therapy can be a valuable tool in treating ASD, it is not a replacement for other forms of therapy or medication when necessary. Play therapy should be used in conjunction with other treatments and under the guidance of a qualified healthcare provider.

In addition, it is important to approach the use of play therapy techniques with sensitivity and respect for the individual needs and preferences of each child with ASD. What works well for one child may not work for another, and therapists must be prepared to adapt and modify their approach as needed to meet the unique needs of each child.

By gaining a better understanding of ASD and the role of play therapy in its treatment, parents and therapists can work together to provide children with ASD the support and resources they need to thrive. The following chapters will provide a comprehensive overview of playful therapy techniques for ASD and the benefits they can offer for children with this complex disorder.

We will also explore some of the challenges and ethical consid- erations that arise when using play therapy techniques in ASD treatment, as well as the professional opportunities available for those that have a keen desire to follow a profession in this particular area.

Overall, the goal of this book is to provide a comprehensive and informative guide to play therapy for autism, offering parents and therapists the tools and knowledge they need to effectively incorporate play into their ASD treatment plan. With the right approach and a commitment to ongoing research and learning, playful therapy has the potential to make a significant difference in the lives of children with ASD and their families.

In the next chapter, we will dive deeper into the benefits of using play therapy in the treatment of ASD and how it can help children with autism develop the skills they need to thrive.

2

The Benefits of Play Therapy for Autism

Play is a natural part of childhood and a crucial tool for children's development. For children with ASD, play therapy can be particularly beneficial, helping to improve communication, socialization, and behavior. Here are some of the key benefits of using play therapy techniques in the treatment of ASD:

1. Improving communication skills

Play therapy can help children with ASD develop their communication skills by providing a safe and fun environment for them to practice social interaction and language. Through play, children can learn to express themselves and understand the perspectives of others.

2. Enhancing socialization

Children with ASD often struggle with socialization, but play therapy can help them develop social skills and build relationships with others. Playful therapy can help children with ASD learn how to initiate and respond to social cues, take turns, and engage in collaborative play.

3. Reducing anxiety and stress

Play therapy can be a source of comfort and relaxation for children with ASD, helping to reduce anxiety and stress. Through play, children can explore their emotions, work through fears and anxieties, and develop coping strategies.

4. Promoting creativity and imagination

Play therapy encourages creativity and imagination, helping children with ASD develop their cognitive skills and problem-solving abilities. Through play, children can explore new ideas, experiment with different approaches, and discover new solutions.

5. Supporting sensory integration

Many children with ASD experience sensory sensitivities, but play therapy can help them learn to regulate their sensory experiences and build their tolerance for different stimuli. Play therapy can involve sensory-based activities, such as sensory bins or play dough, which can help children with ASD develop their sensory processing skills.

Overall, play therapy can be an effective tool for helping children with ASD develop the skills they need to communicate, socialize, and function more effectively. In the following chapters, we will explore specific play therapy techniques and strategies for incorporating play into ASD therapy sessions.

3

Play Therapy Techniques for Autism

There are a variety of play therapy techniques that can be used in the treatment of ASD. Here are some of the most common techniques and strategies:

1. Sensory-based play

Sensory-based play involves using different textures, colors, and smells to help children with ASD develop their sensory processing skills. This can include activities such as playing with play dough, exploring sensory bins, or participating in sensory walks.

2. Pretend play

Pretend play involves using imagination and creativity to create scenarios and stories. This type of play can help children with ASD learn how to take on different perspectives, understand social roles, and practice language and communication skills.

3. Gameplay

Games can be a fun and engaging way for children with ASD to develop their social skills and learn how to take turns and follow rules. Simple board games or card games can be adapted to meet the needs of each child.

4. Art-based play

Art-based play involves using creative expression to explore emotions and develop cognitive skills. Activities such as drawing, painting, and collage-making can help children with ASD build their problem-solving abilities and emotional regulation skills.

5. Movement-based play

Movement-based play involves using physical activity and plays to help children with ASD develop their gross motor skills and coordination. Activities such as dancing, yoga, or obstacle courses can be adapted to meet the needs of each child.

6. Play-based therapy sessions

Play-based therapy sessions involve using play as the primary mode of therapy, with the therapist using play to help the child work through emotional and behavioral issues. Play-based therapy can be particularly effective for children with ASD, as it provides a safe and non-threatening environment for them to express themselves and work through challenges.

These are just a few examples of the many play therapy techniques that can be used in the treatment of ASD. By incorporating play into therapy sessions, therapists and parents can help children with ASD develop the skills they need to communicate, socialize, and function more effectively. In the following chapters, we will explore some of the specific strategies and adaptations that can be made to meet the unique needs of each child with ASD.

4

Adapting Play Therapy Techniques for Children with Autism

When working with children with ASD, it is important to adapt play therapy techniques to meet each child's unique needs and abilities. Here are some strategies for adapting play therapy techniques for children with autism:

1. Create a structured environment

Children with ASD often thrive in structured environments with clear routines and expectations. When incorporating play into therapy sessions, it can be helpful to create a consistent structure and routine, using visual schedules or social stories to help the child understand what to expect.

2. Use visual aids

Many children with ASD benefit from visual aids, such as pictures, charts, or diagrams. Using visual aids can help the child understand the goals and expectations of the therapy session, as well as provide a reference for the activities and games being played.

3. Tailor activities to the child's interests

Children with ASD often have specific interests or obsessions, and incorporating these interests into therapy sessions can be a powerful motivator. Tailoring activities and games to the child's interests can help them engage more fully in the therapy process and build their skills and abilities.

4. Provide clear instructions and feedback

Children with ASD may struggle with understanding and following verbal instructions. When incorporating play into therapy sessions, it is important to provide clear and concise instructions, using visual aids or modeling when necessary. Providing positive feedback and reinforcement can also help encourage the child's participation and progress.

5. Allow for breaks and sensory regulation

Children with ASD may become overwhelmed or overstimulated during therapy sessions. Allowing for breaks and incorporating sensory regulation activities, such as deep breathing or sensory-based play, can help the child regulate their emotions and stay engaged in the therapy process.

By adapting play therapy techniques to meet the unique needs of each child with ASD, therapists, and parents can create a supportive and effective therapy environment. In the following chapters, we will explore specific examples of how play therapy techniques can be adapted for different ages, abilities, and interests.

5

Play Therapy Techniques for Toddlers with Autism

Toddlers with ASD require a specific approach to therapy that incorporates play and sensory-based activities. Here are some examples of playful therapy techniques that can be used with toddlers with autism:

1. Sensory bins

Sensory bins filled with different textures, shapes, and colors can be a fun and engaging way for toddlers with ASD to explore their senses and build their sensory processing skills. Adding toys or objects related to the child's interests can also help them engage more fully in the activity.

2. Bubble play

Blowing bubbles can be a simple but effective way to engage toddlers with ASD in playful therapy. Blowing bubbles can help children develop their breathing and oral motor skills, as well as provide a sensory experience through the tactile sensations of the bubbles.

3. Pretend to play with props

Toddlers with ASD may benefit from using props and toys to engage in pretend play. Using familiar objects, such as toy cars or dolls, can help the child feel more comfortable and confident in their play. Encouraging the child to act out familiar routines, such as mealtime or bedtime, can also help them develop their social skills and language abilities.

4. Music and movement

Music and movement-based play can be a fun and engaging way for toddlers with ASD to build their gross motor skills and co-ordination. Dancing, clapping, or playing musical instruments can help the child develop their rhythm and movement abilities.

5. Visual games

Toddlers with ASD often respond well to visual games and activities that use pictures, charts, or diagrams. Simple matching games or puzzles can help the child develop their cognitive skills and problem-solving abilities.

By incorporating playful therapy techniques into sessions with toddlers with ASD, therapists, and parents can help them develop their skills and abilities in a supportive and engaging environment. By using props, sensory-based activities, and visual aids, therapists can create a fun and interactive therapy experience that meets the unique needs of each child.

6

Play Therapy Techniques for School-Age Children with Autism

School-age children with ASD may require different types of play therapy techniques that build on their social and cognitive skills. Here are some examples of play therapy techniques that can be used with school-age children with autism:

1. Social skills games

Games that focus on building social skills, such as turn-taking and communication, can be helpful for school-age children with ASD. Examples of social skills games include board games, card games, and role-playing activities.

2. Art therapy

Art therapy can be a useful tool for school-age children with ASD, allowing them to express their emotions and develop their creativity. Activities such as drawing, painting, and sculpting can help the child develop their fine motor skills and sensory processing abilities.

3. Lego therapy

Lego therapy is a structured group therapy technique that uses Lego building blocks to help children with ASD develop their social and communication skills. Children work together to build a Lego creation, with each child assigned a specific role, such as "builder," "engineer," or "supplier."

4. Outdoor play

Outdoor play and physical activities, such as playing catch or running races, can be a fun and engaging way for school-age children with ASD to build their gross motor skills and social skills. Outdoor play can also provide a sensory-rich environment that can help the child regulate their emotions and behavior.

5. Video game therapy

Video game therapy uses specially designed video games to help children with ASD develop their cognitive and social skills. Games such as Minecraft and Lego City Undercover allow children to engage in problem-solving and decision-making activities, while also providing a social context for communication and collaboration.

By using a variety of play therapy techniques, therapists and parents can help school-age children with ASD build their social, cognitive, and emotional skills in a fun and engaging way. By focusing on the child's interests and strengths, therapists can create a supportive and effective therapy experience that meets the unique needs of each child.

7

Play Therapy Techniques for Adolescents with Autism

Adolescents with ASD require a different approach to therapy that recognizes their increased independence and autonomy. Here are some examples of play therapy techniques that can be used with adolescents with autism:

1. Role-playing and drama

Role-playing and drama activities can be used to help adolescents with ASD build their social skills and emotional regulation. These activities can also help the child develop their self-expression and communication skills.

2. Video production

Video production can be a fun and engaging way for adolescents with ASD to develop their creativity and social skills. The child can work with others to create a video or short film, learning skills such as scriptwriting, acting, and video editing.

3. Group games

Group games, such as board games, card games, and role-playing games, can help adolescents with ASD develop their social skills, communication, and problem-solving abilities. Games that incorporate strategy and planning can also help the child develop executive functioning skills.

4. Virtual reality therapy

Virtual reality therapy uses virtual reality technology to provide a safe and controlled environment for adolescents with ASD to practice real-world situations. For example, virtual reality therapy can be used to simulate social situations, such as job interviews or public speaking events, allowing the child to practice their social and communication skills in a supportive environment.

5. Sensory-based activities

Adolescents with ASD may still benefit from sensory-based activities, such as sensory bins, textured materials, or fidget toys, to help them regulate their emotions and behavior. These activities can also provide a calming and enjoyable experience for the child.

By using play therapy techniques that recognize the unique needs and abilities of adolescents with ASD, therapists, and parents can help them develop their skills and confidence in a fun and engaging way. By providing opportunities for creative expression, social interaction, and problem-solving, therapists can help adolescents with ASD reach their full potential and lead fulfilling lives.

8

Play Therapy Techniques for Adults with Autism

Play therapy techniques can also be used with adults with ASD to help them develop their social, communication, and self-advocacy skills. Here are some examples of play therapy techniques that can be used with adults with autism:

1. Improv and acting classes

Improv and acting classes can be used to help adults with ASD build their social skills, communication, and emotional regulation. These activities can also help the individual develop self-confidence and creative expression.

2. Board games and puzzles

Board games and puzzles can be a fun and engaging way for adults with ASD to socialize and develop their cognitive skills. Games that involve strategy and planning can also help the individual develop executive functioning skills.

3. Sports and exercise

Sports and exercise can provide a sensory-rich environment that can help adults with ASD regulate their emotions and behavior. Activities such as swimming, yoga, and martial arts can also help the individual develop their physical skills and coordination.

4. Drama therapy

Drama therapy uses theatrical techniques to help adults with ASD develop their social skills, emotional regulation, and self-expression. Activities such as role-playing, improvisation, and storytelling can help individual develop their communication and interpersonal skills.

5. Technology-based activities

Technology-based activities, such as video games, virtual reality, and social media, can provide opportunities for adults with ASD to socialize and connect with others in a safe and controlled environment. These activities can also help the individual develop their digital literacy and technology skills.

By using play therapy techniques that recognize the unique needs and abilities of adults with ASD, therapists, and support workers can help them develop their skills and independence in a fun and engaging way. By providing opportunities for creative expression, social interaction, and problem-solving, adults with ASD can lead fulfilling and meaningful lives.

9

Challenges and Considerations for Play Therapy for Autism

While play therapy can be a powerful tool for individuals with autism, some challenges and considerations must be taken into account. Here are some of the challenges and considerations that therapists and parents should keep in mind when using play therapy for autism:

1. Sensory sensitivity

Individuals with autism may be sensitive to certain sounds, textures, and stimuli, which can make certain play therapy activities challenging or overwhelming. It is important to choose activities that are sensory-friendly and non-threatening.

2. Communication challenges

Individuals with autism may have difficulty communicating their needs, emotions, and preferences. It is important for therapists and parents to use clear and concise language and to be mindful of nonverbal cues.

3. Individualized approach

Autism is a spectrum disorder, and each individual with autism has unique strengths, challenges, and preferences. Therapists and parents need to tailor the playful therapy approach to the individual's specific needs and abilities.

4. Safety considerations

Play therapy activities should be designed with safety in mind, particularly for individuals with autism who may tend to engage in repetitive or impulsive behaviors.

5. Ethical considerations

Play therapy activities should be conducted safely and ethically, with the individual's well-being as the top priority. Therapists and parents should be mindful of ethical guidelines and professional standards when using play therapy for autism.

By being mindful of these challenges and considerations, therapists and parents can ensure that play therapy is used safely and effectively to help individuals with autism develop their skills and reach their full potential.

10

Conclusion

Play therapy is a powerful tool for individuals with autism, providing a fun and engaging way to develop social, communication, and self-advocacy skills. By using play therapy techniques that are tailored to the individual's needs and abilities, therapists and parents can help individuals with autism develop their skills and independence in a meaningful and fulfilling way.

Through activities such as pretend play, sensory play, and social games, individuals with autism can develop their creativity, problem-solving skills, and emotional regulation. By providing a safe and supportive environment for play therapy, therapists and parents can help individuals with autism build self-confidence, improve their social connections, and achieve their goals.

However, it is important to be mindful of the challenges and considerations that come with using play therapy for autism, such as sensory sensitivity, communication challenges, individualized approaches, safety considerations, and ethical considerations. By being aware of these challenges, therapists and parents can ensure that play therapy is used safely and effectively to support the individual's well-being and development.

Overall, play therapy offers a unique and valuable approach to therapy for individuals with autism, providing a fun and engaging way to develop skills, build connections, and achieve their goals. By embracing the power of play, therapists and parents can help individuals with autism reach their full potential and lead fulfilling and meaningful lives.

11

A note of Gratitude to my Readers

Thank you for reading this guide on play therapy for autism. We hope that you have gained a better understanding of how play therapy can be used to support individuals with autism and their families.

Remember, play therapy is just one tool that can be used in the broader landscape of autism therapy and support. It is important to work with qualified professionals, such as licensed therapists and medical providers, to develop a comprehensive treatment plan that meets the individual's unique needs.

If you or someone you know is seeking autism support, there are many resources available, including support groups, advocacy organizations, and educational resources. By working together, we can build a more inclusive and supportive society for individuals with autism and their families.

Thank you for your interest in play therapy for autism, and we wish you all the best in your journey toward health and happiness.

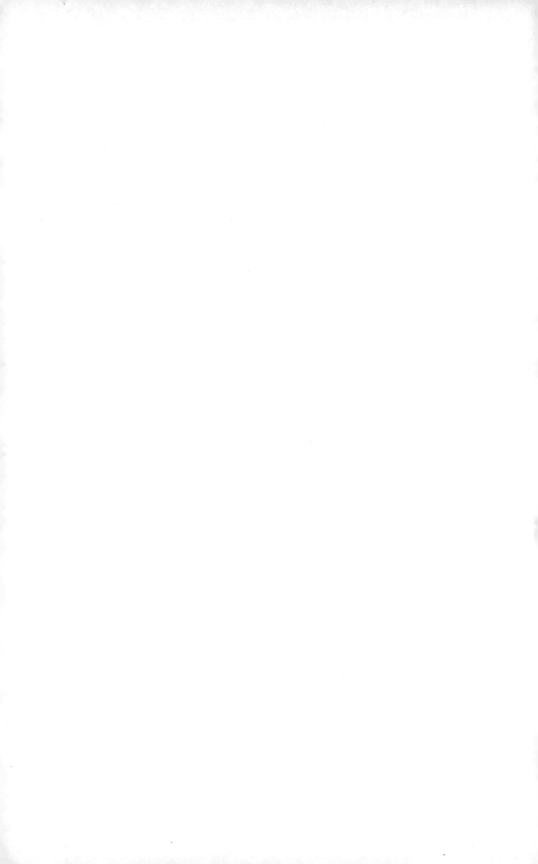

Made in the USA
Las Vegas, NV
14 July 2023

74610758R00022